ADRENAL FATIGUE

Diagnosis and Adrenal Fatigue Tests

Piet Wambacq

Table of Contents

CHAPTER ONE

INRODUCTION

Adrenal Fatigue

- What Is Adrenal Fatigue?

- Symptoms

- Causes

- Treatments

- Risks and Side Effects

Did you know that persistent strain can affect your body's capability to recover from physical, mental or emotional stress? This is probable why the general public have dealt with adrenal fatigue in some unspecified time in the future of their lives.

Many proponents of this circumstance estimate that almost anyone can revel in adrenal fatigue, additionally referred to as hypoadrenia, to a few degree at a especially traumatic point in his or her life.

Because the adrenals affect many elements of the body, signs of adrenal fatigue can mimic some of disorders and isn't usually without problems recognizable.

Adrenal fatigue signs, like brain fog, moodiness and hassle slumbering, may be indicative of many disorders and are often left out via docs. But increasingly more humans are starting to recognize that a combination of these health problems often indicate the onset of adrenal fatigue.

If you've got adrenal fatigue, it could have vast consequences in your overall fitness. Luckily, you may enhance this commonplace issue naturally through focusing in your nutrient consumption and life-style alternatives.

What Is Adrenal Fatigue?

A incredibly new term, "adrenal fatigue" changed into proposed as a new circumstance in 1998 by way of Dr. James L. Wilson, a naturopath and chiropractor. His assumption was that an overstimulation of the adrenal glands (or "adrenals") through lengthy-time period strain may want to lead to an inconsistent level of cortisol (the stress hormone) inside the bloodstream.

In addition to this overload or incorrect pressure hormone ranges, humans with adrenal fatigue frequently don't have enough DHEA, the "figure hormone" answerable for the advent of many important hormones in the body.

The unique progression of adrenal fatigue all through the day as follows:

- You wake up and are unable to function without a good sized quantity of caffeine.

- You eventually experience a lift of electricity for the duration of the early a part of the day.

- Then your electricity levels crash round 2 p.M., upward push around 6 p.M. And fall once more round nine p.M.

- Your electricity finally peaks again at 11 p.M.

Is Adrenal Fatigue Real?

The primary difficulty with recognizing or diagnosing

adrenal fatigue is the inability to differentiate its signs and patterns from different problems. The parameters for this condition are nonspecific, which, regrettably, has brought about a amazing controversy around this subject matter, even though the very nature of cortisol and physical hormones is that the results are far-attaining.

A diagnosis for this circumstance is tough because pressure hormone degrees typically fall in what conventional medicinal drug would call "in the ordinary range," although the signs are clean to those affected by the condition.

People who believe that adrenal fatigue isn't a actual health difficulty often kingdom that constant ranges of continual strain haven't any impact on the adrenals and the most effective authentic endocrine problems are the ones resulting from other diseases and direct harm to the adrenal glands.

However, many practitioners of natural medicine recognize, from experience in a health care exercise and supporting medical proof, that hypoadrenia may be very actual and related to some of complications.

In addition, adrenal fatigue treatment is enormously noninvasive and is useful on your health, irrespective of the diagnosis. Of course, you must be beneath the care of a certified clinical professional, consisting of a practical medicinal drug health practitioner, you agree with, and notice her or him about any signs and symptoms you enjoy (of any disorder) so the medical doctor can determine appropriate remedy.

CHAPTER TWO

The Adrenal Glands

Your adrenal glands (adrenals) are thumb-sized organs that sit down above your kidneys and are a part of the endocrine gadget. Also called the suprarenal glands, they're worried in producing over 50 hormones that power almost each bodily feature, a lot of which might be vital for existence.

The adrenal glands paintings carefully with the hypothalamus and the pituitary gland in a system known as the hypothalamus-pituitary-adrenal axis (HPA axis).

Adrenal glands play a large position in strain response. Here's how it works:

•   Your mind registers a danger, whether emotional, intellectual or bodily.

•   The adrenal medulla releases cortisol and adrenaline hormones that will help you react to the chance (the fight-or-flight response), rushing blood for your brain, coronary heart and muscle groups.

•   The adrenal cortex then releases corticosteroids to dampen approaches like digestion, immune gadget reaction and different features no longer important for immediate survival.

Your adrenal glands are also accountable for balancing hormones.

Problems with Adrenal Function

When discussing problems with adrenal feature, it's vital to understand that adrenal fatigue is not the identical element as adrenal insufficiency, Addison's sickness or Cushing's syndrome/Cushing's ailment.

Here's a short breakdown of these conditions and how they

are one of a kind than adrenal fatigue:

Adrenal Insufficiency and Addison's disease:

•	Symptoms found in adrenal insufficiency that aren't found in adrenal fatigue include principal digestive troubles, weight reduction, low blood sugar, headache and sweating.

•	Primary adrenal insufficiency is what's referred to as Addison's disease and happens whilst the adrenal glands are damaged by using some kind of trauma and may't produce sufficient cortisol or aldosterone.

- Secondary adrenal insufficiency (that is greater commonplace) occurs when the pituitary gland stops generating adrenocorticotropin (ACTH). ACTH is what stimulates the adrenal glands to provide cortisol.

- What differentiates this condition from adrenal fatigue? More often than now not, adrenal fatigue is modeled by way of an overabundance of strain hormone ranges, frequently at the "incorrect" instances, even as adrenal insufficiency is a regular incapacity to produce cortisol.

- •   The biggest difference among them is that people with adrenal fatigue usually have cortisol ranges that fall in "ordinary" levels but now not "optimum," while adrenal insufficiency sufferers have cortisol degrees continually outdoor the ordinary variety.

Cushing's Syndrome/Disease:

- •   Cushing's disorder is an exceptionally uncommon disease that includes the overproduction of cortisol, outdoor the regular stages, that most often influences girls among 25–forty.

- •   This situation is sometimes the end result of tumors, and in different instances, there may be no acknowledged reason.

- Cushing's may be reversed and is defined as a "curable" condition with the aid of the National Institute of Health.

- Unique signs and symptoms of Cushing's syndrome (referred to as Cushing's ailment when resulting from a pituitary tumor) consist of stomach/facial weight benefit, male impotence, failure to menstruate, increased danger of miscarriage, high blood sugar and excessive blood stress.

Symptoms

What occurs whilst the adrenal glands forestall producing hormones correctly?

Every bodily function is affected, and as adrenal hormone degrees ebb and glide abnormally, even the regular "get-up-and-move" you get from them disappears.

Adrenal fatigue symptoms encompass:

•	Autoimmune situations

•	Chronic fatigue (always feeling worn-out)

•	Brain fog

•	Hair loss

- Hormone imbalance

- Weakened strain response

- Insulin resistance

- Lightheadedness

- Decreased intercourse power/libido

- Moodiness and irritability

- Depression

- Muscle or bone loss

- Skin ailments

- Sleep disturbances/sleep apnea

- Weight advantage

- Sweet and salty food cravings

- Loss of appetite

As you can see, there are a number of signs that is probably related to different underlying problems, which include some very commonplace women's health issues.

Fortunately, the approaches to fight those problems are very similar and benefit your overall health. If you've skilled any of these adrenal fatigue aspect effects, take coronary heart, for there are actually many natural approaches to treat and guide your adrenal gadget.

Causes

Adrenal fatigue is a condition in which the frame and adrenal glands can't hold up with the extremely good amount of day by day pressure many humans revel in. Sometimes misunderstood as an autoimmune ailment, adrenal fatigue can mimic a few precursors to different not unusual ailments and diseases.

Wellness medical doctors and practitioners believe that an episode of acute pressure or extended (mainly for over a 12 months), ongoing stress can purpose adrenal glands to end up overloaded and ineffective, then improperly launch cortisol. They accept as true with that hypoadrenia can be due to:

•	Stressful stories like death of loved one, divorce or surgical procedure

•	Exposure to environmental toxins and pollutants

•	Prolonged strain because of monetary difficulty, horrific relationships or work environment, and other conditions that entail emotions of helplessness

•	Negative wondering and emotional trauma

•	Lack of sleep

•	Poor weight loss plan (together with crash diets and

inconsistent nutrition) and shortage of workout

• Pain

• Food sensitivities

• Adverse events in childhood

• Surgery

• Reliance on stimulants like caffeine or energy beverages

• Rheumatoid arthritis

• Diabetes/impaired glucose levels

Can strain purpose extreme fatigue? Yes, it virtually can.

One examine located that scholars undergoing chronic, lengthy-time period pressure whilst prepping for medical assessments on the cease in their academic careers impaired the students' cortisol awakening reaction.

By restricting this surge in cortisol that clearly occurs every morning whilst you wake up that will help you sense alert, strain inhibits your ability to wake up absolutely, irrespective of how tons sleep you get.

Another examine, released in 2005, found that students diagnosed with continual fatigue syndrome had "changes in adrenal characteristic," in particular in ladies, suggesting that their adrenal glands were not receiving a normal amount of stimulation.

Depression may play a position inside the improvement or effects of adrenal fatigue. Research suggests that once a prime depressive episode, cortisol responses do not without difficulty readjust to regular degrees and is probably incredibly responsible for a recurrence of despair.

And there's research suggesting that hypothalamic disorder is commonplace in a couple of sclerosis, an autoimmune sickness. Researchers are comparing why dysfunction of the hypothalamic-pituitary-adrenal axis is not unusual in multiple sclerosis, but it's believed to be connected to strange cortisol secretion.

CHAPTER THREE

TREATMENTS

There are both traditional and natural remedies for adrenal fatigue. The first step is to diagnose the hassle, which may be hard due to the fact the general public pass too lengthy truly handling their signs and symptoms.

Diagnosis and Adrenal Fatigue Tests

Many human beings go for some time without consulting their standard physicians or endocrinologists about some of the signs of adrenal fatigue. This is one foremost motive why diagnosis of this condition is unusual.

However, experiencing excessive cortisol symptoms over an extended period of time can certainly take a toll. In addition, a few signs can be indicative of greater serious conditions.

If you enjoy one or a mixture of adrenal fatigue signs for an extended time period and your symptoms have all started interfering with regular existence, relationships and/or sports — such as work, family time or college — it's time to visit your medical doctor and ask about adrenal fatigue.

Adrenal Fatigue Tests

Tests for adrenal fatigue are, unluckily, any other supply of bewilderment for lots. You need to know in advance of time that these assessments should be accomplished via someone who knows the nature of adrenal fatigue and that exams for adrenal fatigue are not often definitive.

The most commonplace of these tests includes trying out physical fluid for cortisol. Blood tests are almost by no means helpful on this regard, but a 24-hour salivary panel may help your doctor understand peculiar cortisol styles, together with an absence or overload of pressure response.

Many medical doctors additionally check thyroid function alongside cortisol ranges because of the manner these hormonal structures are interconnected.

Other exams that may be used to help diagnose or verify adrenal fatigue consist of:

• ACTH Challenge

• TSH takes a look at (thyroid stimulating hormone)

• Free T3 (FT3)

• Total Thyroxine (TT4)

• Cortisol/DHEA ratio

- 17-HP/Cortisol ratio

- Neurotransmitter trying out

There are also safe home assessments you could strive, which include:

- The Iris Contraction Test: The principle at the back of this take a look at is that the iris will now not have the ability to properly contract while exposed to light in humans with weakened adrenal feature. The test involves sitting in a dark room and shining a flashlight in brief across the eyes repeatedly. If you have adrenal fatigue, it's possible that the eye contraction will ultimate no extra than two minutes and the eyes will dilate even if nonetheless exposed to direct light

• Postural Low Blood Pressure Test: In healthy individuals, blood strain rises when growing from a laying role. Using a blood stress monitor, you may take a look at your stress while laying down after which after standing. If you notice no rise or a drop in your tiers, it's possible your adrenals had been weakened.

Conventional Treatment

Because of the debatable nature of this condition, you

could need to are trying to find out a naturopath who will help you treat adrenal fatigue with a combination of dietary advice and complement pointers, in addition to any hormonal or different medications important.

Studies imply that an oral dose of 20 milligrams of hydrocortisone is recommended with the aid of some for recurring cortisol control, even as an occasional dose of 50 milligrams may be prescribed however ought to now not be taken frequently or in higher doses.

Your physician or endocrinologist should assist you apprehend the ability side effects of this and some other medicinal drug encouraged.

CHAPTER FOUR

NATURAL TREATMENTS

Treatment for adrenal fatigue involves:

•	lowering stress on your body and your thoughts

•	casting off toxins

•	avoiding terrible thinking

•	replenishing your body with healthy foods, dietary supplements and methods of thinking

If you're asking, "How can I assist my adrenal glands?" the answer may be closer than you watched adrenal fatigue remedy appears plenty just like the healthy, recuperation diets to assist fight the underlying troubles inflicting a number of situations.

1. Follow the Adrenal Fatigue Diet

In every case of adrenal recuperation, diet is a big thing. There are a number of foods that provide adrenal help, supporting replenish your adrenal energy so your system can come back to complete health.

First, you must start by putting off any hard-to-digest meals and any pollutants or chemical compounds for your environment.

The idea behind the adrenal fatigue weight loss program is to get rid of some thing that taxes your adrenals.

Foods to avoid encompass:

•	Caffeine: Caffeine can intrude together with your sleep cycle and make it hard to your adrenals to recover. If you ought to drink espresso or a caffeinated beverage, then have a restricted quantity in the morning earlier than noon.

•	Sugar and sweeteners: Try to keep away from as a whole lot extra sugar as feasible. This consists of avoiding excessive-fructose corn syrup and synthetic sweeteners as nicely. Avoid sugary ingredients, cereals, candy and chocolates. Be aware that sugar is an additive in lots of breads, condiments and dressings. Seek uncooked honey or stevia as options, and continually moderate your use of sweeteners of any kind.

•   Carbohydrates: While carbohydrates aren't all horrific for you, the inflammation they are able to motive is especially difficult whilst experiencing adrenal fatigue. Many people crave carb-heavy meals after they're careworn, which provide a non permanent pride however end up taxing the adrenal glands more. If you're overwhelmed and burdened out, try kicking the gluten and starchy carbs for a time period to see if which could modify your tiredness and power degrees.

•   Processed and microwaved foods: First of all, the microwave has its personal risks, but moreover, maximum microwaveable, ultra-processed ingredients have many preservatives and fillers which are tough to digest and put on out your frame's power and digestion cycle. Try to shop for meals at the outer walls of your grocery store, and put together your personal meals on every occasion feasible.

- Processed meats: An overload of protein can stress your hormones more than you may assume, and the added hormones and lacking vitamins in conventional, processed meats (specifically purple meats like beef and steak) can throw your device out of whack in quick succession. When shopping for meats for adrenal aid, stick to grass-fed red meat and unfastened-range fowl or turkey, and devour these protein-heavy meats handiest moderately.

- Hydrogenated oils: Vegetable oils like soybean, canola and corn oil are notably inflammatory and can lead to adrenal inflammation. Try to simplest use top fats which include coconut oil, olive oil, organic butter or ghee.

Next, you need to feature nutrient-dense meals which might be clean to digest and have recuperation characteristics.

Foods to feature on your weight loss program include:

- Coconut

- Olives

- Avocado and other healthful fats

- Cruciferous vegetables (cauliflower, broccoli, Brussels sprouts, and so forth.)

- Fatty fish (e.G., wild-caught salmon)

- Free-variety fowl and turkey

- Bone broth

- Nuts, together with walnuts and almonds

- Seeds, which include pumpkin, chia and flax

- Kelp and seaweed

- Celtic or Himalayan sea salt

•	Fermented meals rich in probiotics

•	Chaga and cordyceps medicinal mushrooms

These meals help triumph over adrenal fatigue because they're nutrient-dense, low in sugar and feature healthy fats and fiber.

2. Supplements and Herbs

Another major trade to overcoming adrenal fatigue is taking the proper dietary supplements the usage of supporting herbs. Because it can nevertheless be an undertaking to get enough of every nutrient you want every day, supplements may be used to make certain that you get the nutrients and minerals which might be important for adrenal guide.

In addition, there are certain herbs, spices and essential oils which could assist to fight adrenal fatigue and help an active, vibrant existence.

•	Adaptogenic herbs ashwagandha, rhodiola rosea, schisandra and holy basil. By the usage of these herbs in food coaching, you could alleviate a number of the strain in your adrenal glands.

•	Licorice root: This spice is available in extract shape and has been shown to help boom the DHEA to your body. Licorice root is associated with a few aspect results and may from time to time be avoided with the aid of taking DGL licorice. Research suggests that pregnant ladies and those with heart, liver or kidney problems need to avoid licorice root. Don't take it for extra than four weeks at a time. Make sure to display blood stress, as ranges can boom in a few sufferers.

• Fish oil (EPA/DHA): There is a huge quantity of advantages of supplementing with fish oil (or, for humans on vegan or different plant-based diets, algal oil). Several of those consist of counteracting some of adrenal fatigue-associated symptoms and headaches, consisting of diabetes, mental dysfunction, arthritis, immune gadget function, skin problems, gaining weight and anxiety/despair.

•   Magnesium: Magnesium is one of the important vitamins for fighting adrenal insufficiency. While the mechanisms of this aren't absolutely understood, you may gain from supplementing with magnesium in case you are affected by adrenal fatigue.

•   B-Complex nutrients: Research finds that vitamin B12 deficiency can be associated with strain on the adrenal cortex in some animals. Vitamin B5 is another commonly poor vitamin in human beings with adrenal pressure. Especially in case you're lowering or casting off meat from your weight-reduction plan on the way to fight adrenal fatigue, it can serve you well to take a splendid B-complex nutrition complement.

• Vitamin C: Known as a "strain-busting" nutrient, nutrition C seems to limit the outcomes of stress on people as well as lessen the time vital to get better from worrying activities.

• Vitamin D: In addition to maintaining homeostasis between magnesium and phosphorus within the body and assisting strong bones, diet D may also effect other conditions, including adrenal dysfunction and disease.

•	Selenium: At least one animal look at finds that selenium deficiency can negatively affect adrenal feature.

•	Lavender oil: Human and animal studies display that lavender critical oil has a chilled impact that could reduce strain. Research additionally indicates that it is able to lower excessive cortisol tiers when inhaled.

- Rosemary oil: Rosemary important oil (along side lavender) may additionally decrease cortisol concentrations and reduce oxidative strain on cells.

Remember to use entire-food-based dietary supplements from legitimate companies, and use most effective a hundred percent, therapeutic-grade, USDA Certified Organic important oils. Make certain you trust what you buy.

3. Reduce Stress

The maximum vital key to restoring your adrenal characteristic is to heed your thoughts and strain wishes.

CHAPTER SIX

PAY ATTENTION TO YOUR FRAME, AND TRY THE SUBSEQUENT NATURAL STRESS RELIEVERS:

1.   Rest while you feel tired as much as feasible.

2.   Sleep 8–10 hours a 19.

3.   Avoid staying up late and stay on a normal sleep cycle — ideally, in bed earlier than 10 p.M.

4.   Laugh and do something amusing every day.

5.   Minimize work and relational strain however possible.

6.   Eat on a regular food cycle, and decrease your caffeine and sugar addiction.

7.   Exercise (even slight exercise and on foot can help). Yoga, specially, can help to enhance first-rate of lifestyles and reduce stress responses. If you feel worn-out after exercise, it's once in a while beneficial to most effective walk till adrenals are sufficiently healed.

8.   Avoid negative people and self-talk.

9.   Take time for yourself (do something enjoyable).

10.   Seek suggest or help for any stressful experiences.

Let's talk about "self-speak" for a minute. Our bodies are made to heal. However, the phrases we are saying have a terrific impact on our body and our ability to heal.

Regardless of what weight-reduction plan and dietary supplements you take, your surroundings are one of the maximum important additives.

So, be kind to yourself. Try to avoid pronouncing terrible matters about yourself and others. It's essential to choose to be around positive humans and live advantageous approximately yourself as well.

Many people roll their eyes at such recommendation, however it's scientifically verified that it's feasible to reduce pathological worry with the aid of training "thought replacement," a tremendous self-communicate practice that involves verbally reciting nice results to worrying conditions.

4. Recovery

How long does it take to recover? It's not an clean query to reply because adrenal fatigue recuperation time has by no means been studied.

Recovery for adrenal fatigue can take a little while, even

though. After all, it took months, maybe years, to wear out your adrenals — so it takes a bit times to accumulate their power once more.

For full adrenal healing, you can expect it to take:

•	6–9 months for minor adrenal fatigue

•	12–18 months for moderate fatigue

•	Up to 24 months for intense adrenal fatigue

The pleasant approach is to make solid changes in your life-style for lasting effects. Some people word a distinction of their standard nicely-being after only some weeks of better foods that aid in detoxification of the frame and adrenal fatigue supplements.

If you aim for a balanced life-style with a healthy level of sleep, exercise, amusing and a wonderful environment, then you definately are most probably to hold your adrenal gadget going sturdy!

Risks and Side Effect

First, understand that any new dietary regimen or addition of supplements to your way of life must be implemented underneath the supervision of a physician/naturopath you consider.

 In widespread, introducing greater plant-primarily based foods into your lifestyle and disposing of stimulants, sugary foods and processed gadgets with a ton of sodium or chemical substances delivered to them goes that will help you sense and live higher, no matter situations you can or may not have.

The larger subject comes while referring to herbs, spices, dietary supplements and critical oils used to combat adrenal fatigue. Don't blindly use any new dietary supplements, herb or vital oil without scientific supervision or proper schooling on how, how a lot, how often and how lengthy to apply these dietary supplements.

There are numerous herbs that have to now not be used when pregnant or breastfeeding. This consists of medicinal mushrooms, adaptogenic herbs and some essential oils.

Final Thoughts

• Adrenal fatigue is a controversial condition taken into consideration to be an "in-between" nation of fitness, before achieving a nation of diagnosable disorder.

- It's stated to be due to high degrees of chronic stress that lead to a taxing of the adrenal glands, forcing them to overproduce or underproduce cortisol, the stress hormone, at the incorrect instances.

- Common signs of adrenal fatigue consist of intense tiredness, brain fog, decreased sex pressure, hair loss, insulin resistance and others.

- To certainly combat adrenal fatigue, do away with inflammatory ingredients out of your weight loss plan including sugar and extra carbohydrates, and devour lots of colourful, plant-primarily based foods, free-variety lean meats including chook or turkey, and lots of healthy fats.

•	There are a variety of herbs, spices, dietary supplements and crucial oils that can be used to combat adrenal fatigue. These ought to be used below scientific supervision.

THE END

www.ingramcontent.com/pod-product-compliance
Lightning Source LLC
Chambersburg PA
CBHW060842260726
48661CB00002B/568